Runners Replenish

Nutritional and Fitness Lessons from Top Athletes

Table of Contents

Chapter 1. Introduction

Welcome to "Runners Replenish: Nutritional and Fitness Lessons from Top Athletes"! This specially curated report brings together essential insights about nutrition and fitness from some of the world's leading runners. Uncover the secrets that fuel their stamina, delve into their carefully crafted diet plans, and uncover the unique fitness strategies that build their speed and agility. Our special report is no less than a treasure chest of precious knowledge for both aspiring runners and seasoned athletes. Written in an engaging and approachable style, you'll find it fascinating, practical, and absolutely indispensable. Unwrap this bundle of wisdom from the best in the field and step up your running game. You're just one read away from powering your performance and crossing your next finish line faster and stronger than ever before!

Chapter 2. Defining the Runner's Diet: Essential Nutrients and Macros

There's a popular saying among runners that you can't outrun a bad diet. That's because the food you consume is the fuel for your body - it powers your muscles, feeds your brain, and replenishes nutrients lost through exertion and sweat. But what constitutes the ideal runner's diet? This chapter will break down what you need to know about essential nutrients and macros for runners. Let's dive in!

2.1. Nutrition: More Than Just Energy

Nutrition is about more than just energy. Although carbohydrates, proteins, and fats (the three macronutrients) provide the calories your body needs to function, they also play other specific roles. Carbohydrates are your body's preferred source of fuel, especially for high-intensity exercise. Proteins are necessary for building and repairing muscles, especially after a hard workout. Fats, meanwhile, are important for overall health and can serve as a fuel source for long, slow runs.

Eating a balance of these macronutrients is a key part of a runner's diet. It's also important to include a variety of foods to ensure you get all the necessary micronutrients - vitamins and minerals that your body needs in small quantities - to keep every system in your body working as it should.

2.2. Carbohydrates: A Runner's Best Friend

As a runner, carbohydrates should make up about 60% of your diet. This is because when you eat carbohydrates, your body breaks them down into glucose, a simple sugar, that can be used immediately for energy or stored in your muscles and liver for later use. This stored glucose, called glycogen, is what your body relies on for energy during longer runs.

When training for longer distances or races, a diet high in carbohydrates helps to ensure those glycogen stores are filled to the brim. That's why you'll often hear about runners "carb-loading" before a big race - they're trying to cram as much glycogen into their muscles as possible.

Fiber, a type of carbohydrate found in whole foods like fruits, vegetables, and whole grains, is also crucial. It aids in digestion and helps to keep you feeling full.

2.3. Protein: Building Block of Muscles

Protein should make up about 15-20% of a runner's diet. It's a key player in building and repairing muscle, which is especially important as intensive running can lead to muscle damage. Protein also benefits runners by aiding in recovery, supporting immune function, and promoting the feeling of fullness.

The exact amount of protein you need will depend on your weight and the intensity of your running. A good ballpark figure to aim for is 0.6 to 0.9 grams of protein per pound of body weight.

Good sources of protein for runners include lean meats, fish, eggs, dairy, nuts, and legumes.

2.4. Fats: Slow-Burning Fuel

The remaining 20-30% of a runner's diet should come from fats. Fats are a concentrated source of calories, providing more than double the amount per gram compared to carbohydrates and protein. They are an important fuel source for long, slow runs and also assist in the absorption of fat-soluble vitamins like A, D, E, and K.

It's crucial, however, to focus on the right kinds of fats. Saturated and trans fats, found in things like full-fat dairy, fried foods, and many packaged foods, can lead to heart disease and other health problems. Instead, opt for healthy fats found in foods like avocados, nuts, seeds, olive oil, and fatty fish.

2.5. Vitamins and Minerals: Small but Mighty

Along with these macronutrients, a runner's diet needs to be rich in certain vitamins and minerals - the micronutrients - that play a key role in energy production, bone health, hydration, and muscle function.

Key vitamins and minerals for runners include calcium and vitamin D for bone health; B-vitamins (like thiamin, riboflavin, and niacin) and iron for energy production; sodium, potassium, and chloride for maintaining fluid balance; and magnesium for muscle function.

Remember, a good diet that includes a variety of foods and covers all the macro and micronutrients will always trump relying on supplements.

2.6. Timing Your Nutrient Intake

But it's not just what you eat, it's also when you eat. Timing nutrient intake around workouts can have a big impact on performance and recovery.

As a general rule, try to eat a meal rich in carbs and protein 2-4 hours before a run. If you can't manage a full meal, a smaller snack or drink with a good balance of carbs and protein - think a fruit smoothie with Greek yogurt - can work in a pinch.

Immediately after a run is also a crucial time for refueling. Aim for a snack or meal with a 3:1 carb-to-protein ratio within 30 minutes of finishing your workout to replenish glycogen stores and kickstart muscle recovery.

THE END of this chapter. In the next chapters, we will take a deeper dive into each of these components of a runner's diet, and provide practical advice on how and what to eat to keep your energy levels high, your muscles strong, and your running performance at its peak. Get ready to fuel your running like never before!

Chapter 3. Meal Timing: Pre-Run and Post-Run Feeding Strategies

Fueling your body at the right time is a critical aspect of a successful running routine. Therefore, understanding meal timing – specifically pre-run and post-run feeding strategies – can be instrumental for both performance and recovery phases.

3.1. The Pre-Run Preparation

Your pre-run meal is the fuel that drives your body during intense runs. Understanding the composition of this meal and when to consume it is crucial for maintaining optimal energy levels.

3.1.1. When to Eat Before a Run

As a general rule, larger meals should be eaten three to four hours before a run, allowing your body enough time to digest the food and convert it into useful energy. If you're having a smaller snack, one to two hours before the start works best. Eating too close to a run can lead to gastrointestinal distress, something no runner wants to face mid-run.

3.1.2. What to Eat Before a Run

Carbohydrates are king when it comes to pre-run food. They are your body's preferred energy source, especially for endurance exercises like long-distance running. Aim for complex carbohydrates, as they release energy slowly and provide a steady fuel source. Excellent choices are whole grains, fruits, and vegetables.

However, balance your meal by adding moderate amounts of protein for muscle health and minimal fats, as they might slow digestion. A bowl of oatmeal with berries, banana, and a sprinkle of chia seeds could be a great pre-run meal.

3.2. The Importance of Hydration

Staying well-hydrated cannot be stressed enough in running. Dehydration can impair performance and, in severe instances, can be life-threatening. But when and what should you be drinking?

3.2.1. Hydrating Before a Run

Drink plenty of fluids throughout the day, not only in the hours leading to your run. Consider sipping on a sports drink that contains electrolytes if you plan on running for more than 60 minutes. This helps balance the electrolytes lost through sweat.

3.2.2. Hydrating During and After a Run

If you're running for less than an hour, water should suffice. However, for longer runs, a sports drink containing carbohydrates and electrolytes is advisable to replace what you're losing. Post-run, hydrate with water or drinks with electrolytes, especially if you've completed a long or particularly sweaty run.

3.3. The Post-Run Reward

Post-run nutrition is your opportunity to reward your body for a job well done. Not only will these nutritious meals replenish lost nutrients, they will also help speed up recovery.

3.3.1. When to Eat After a Run

Try to consume a meal or snack within 45 minutes after finishing your run. This window is when your body is primed to replenish energy stores and repair and build muscle tissues.

3.3.2. What to Eat After a Run

A mix of carbohydrates and protein in a 3:1 or 4:1 ratio helps replenish energy stores and repairs muscles. Aim for high-quality proteins and carbs. Foods like quinoa, brown rice, lean meats, eggs, and cottage cheese are popular post-run meals. Don't forget to incorporate fruits and vegetables to provide necessary vitamins and minerals.

3.4. Fueling for Evening Runs

Meal timing for night runners may require additional tricks. Consume a balanced meal with carbs, proteins, and a little healthy fat three to four hours before your run. Around an hour before, you can go for an easily digestible snack. A small post-run meal or snack will ensure your energy stores are filled back up before you sleep.

3.5. Mastering Your Personal Timing

Each runner's body responds differently to food and meal timing. Experiment with different types and amounts of food and find your comfortable pre and post-run nutrition routine.

Keeping a nutrition journal can help you identify trends and correlations between what (and when) you eat and how you perform or recover. As with all aspects of training, patience and consistency are key to nailing your meal timing. Start by incorporating these guidelines into your running routine.

Understanding the nuances of meal timing before and after running can take you up the ladder of performance. It's all about knowing your body and providing it with what it needs, when it needs it. Proper pre and post-run nutrition will help you go farther, recover faster, and prevent injuries - giving you an undeniable edge in your running goals.

Chapter 4. Hydration Habits of Elite Runners

Hydration is a fundamental aspect for any type of athlete, but it carries special importance for long distance runners who sweat profusely during grueling hours on the track. Proper hydration ensures efficient energy utilization, levels optimal body temperature, and maintains muscle activity. This is why world-class runners pay special attention to their hydration routine, making it strategic. Here is an exhaustive depiction of the hydration habits of elite runners.

4.1. Understanding Hydration

Stepping into the subject matter, let's delve into what hydration is and why it's an inseparable part of athletic performance. Our bodies are approximately 60% water, which regulates our temperature and aids in crucial functions such as nutrient transportation, digestion, and joint lubrication. When water level drops, the heart pumps harder to circulate blood, leading to dehydration, which can cause dizziness, fatigue, and even cardiac distress.

Runners may lose up to 3 liters of sweat in an hour. Precise hydration is needed to replace this loss, without causing water intoxication (extreme over-hydration). This fluid balance is mastered by elite runners, comprising timing, type and intake quantity of fluids for optimal performance and recovery.

4.2. Pre-Run Hydration

Every professional runner maintains a disciplined hydration regime before their running sessions. Dehydration, even as slight as 2%, has been scientifically proven to hinder performance. Stamina dips, perceptual awareness blurs, and the body is more prone to injury and cramps.

Mirroring the strategies of elite runners, it's advisable to practice "preloading". This involves consuming 500-1000 mL of fluid (preferably with a small amount of sodium) in the couple of hours before the run. The sodium aids in retaining the fluid, supplying it gradually throughout the run.

4.3. Mid-Run Hydration

Staying hydrated during the run is of utmost importance. A rule of thumb to determine fluid needs is to consider environmental conditions and individual sweating rates.

Elite athletes adopt the 'weigh-test' approach. They weigh themselves before and after workouts to calculate the differential, and then drink 1.25-1.5 L of fluid for each kg lost. During a marathon, runners' options may be limited by the provision of water stations. In lesser controlled circumstances, they bring their own fluids. Generally, a mix of water and sports drinks, which contains electrolytes and carbohydrates, is preferred.

An important note is to listen to your body's signals. Over-hydration, called hyponatremia, can lead to potentially life-threatening situations. Consuming fluids only when thirsty usually works well for runners.

4.4. Post-Run Hydration

Rehydrating post-run is as critical as staying hydrated during the run. It expedites recovery and helps compensate for fluid loss. Runners usually drink a concoction of water and carbohydrate-protein drinks to help restore muscles and replenish glycogen stores. Endurance athletes understand that this post-exercise rehydration permits efficient recovery and long-lasting performance in training or competition.

4.5. Hydrating Foods

Hydration isn't just about drinking fluids. It's also about eating right. Many fruits and vegetables have high water content and provide natural sugars, electrolytes, and fibers. Watermelon, cucumbers, oranges, and strawberries are good examples. Elite runners incorporate such hydrating foods in their diet, which aid in fluid intake.

4.6. Adjusting Hydration for Weather Conditions

Weather conditions play a significant role in hydration strategy. In hotter climates, the fluid and electrolyte loss is more significant, requiring runners to increase their intake. During colder periods, runners must be mindful not to overlook hydration due to less perceived exertion. Each condition requires alteration in hydration plans, a skill that sets champion runners apart.

4.7. Importance of Electrolytes

Apart from water, electrolytes like sodium and potassium are vital. Sodium minimizes urine output and stimulates thirst, thus aiding in fluid balance. Potassium works with sodium to maintain water balance across cell membranes. Therefore, electrolyte-infused drinks are often preferred over regular water.

Hydration isn't a one-size-fits-all technique. It relies heavily on understanding your body's needs, experimenting and refining your approach. Though we bring you an overarching idea of hydration, any comprehensive strategy must be tailored and personalised to match the individual's physiology and ambition. This deep focus on individualised planning is what sets elite runners a stride ahead in performance.

Chapter 5. Training Like a Pro: Practical Workout Plans

As an aspiring runner or a seasoned athlete, it's crucial to understand that every successful running strategy is built upon a robust training plan. Training like a pro implies specificity, consistency, and intensity. Let's explore how these paradigms can translate into realistic, powerful, and efficient workout plans.

5.1. The Importance of Specificity

Specificity refers to identifying and training towards your running goal. Whether it's improving your speed, increasing your endurance, or setting a new personal record – your training should reflect your objective. Consider the terrain, the distance, and the speed at which you'll run, and tailor your workout plan accordingly.

For instance, if you're focusing on running a 10k, your training plan should include specific runs that push you to run that distance or slightly more. You can also incorporate speed workouts that help your body get familiar with the race pace. Moreover, if the race involves uphill running, incorporate hill-repeats in your training to mimic the terrain.

5.2. Consistency is Key

The secret to becoming a pro lies in the consistency of your workouts. This not only involves running regularly but also following a balanced training plan to avoid overloading certain muscle groups while ignoring the others.

Every well-rounded running program must have a blend of long runs for endurance, speed workouts for improving pace, strength training for muscle development and injury prevention, and recovery runs to allow your body to recuperate. Varying your intensity and type of workout during the week can help you maintain a consistent training rhythm.

One sample week of a balanced, consistent training plan might look like this:

```
|===
| Day | Workout

| Monday | Rest or cross-training

| Tuesday | Speed work: 8x400m repeats at fast pace with
jogging recovery in-between

| Wednesday | Easy 5km run + strength training

| Thursday | Long slow run: 10km at easy pace

| Friday | Recovery run: 3-5km at easy pace or rest

| Saturday | Hill repeats: 6x200m uphill at fast pace

| Sunday | Long run: 12-15km at easy to moderate pace
|===
```

5.3. Intensity Matters

It's a common misconception amongst amateur runners that running harder every day will result in faster improvements. Pros know that the secret to better performance is not about running hard, but running smart.

Learning to manage the intensity of your workouts is crucial. You should aim to do 80% of your runs at a low intensity to maintain a strong aerobic base. The remaining 20% can be allocated to high-intensity workouts, such as speed work or hill repeats.

Another useful approach is to use Rate of Perceived Exertion (RPE) to determine the intensity of your workouts. This is a simple way to listen to your body and modify your workouts, depending on how hard you feel you are working.

5.4. Recovery Is Part of Training

Recognize that rest and recovery are part of your training plan. After high-intensity workouts or long runs, your body needs time to replace energy stores, repair damaged tissues, and adapt to the stress of the workout. Without adequate recovery, your body will not be able to reap the full benefits of the training, leading to stagnation or injuries.

Recovery can be passive — such as taking a full rest day, getting quality sleep, or opting for light activities such as walking or yoga. Or it can be active — such as easy recovery runs, cross-training activities, or functional body exercises that facilitate blood circulation and tissue repair.

5.5. Embrace Strength Training

Strength training may not seem directly related to running faster or further, but it plays an invaluable role in boosting overall running performance. It helps build stronger muscles, bones, tendons, and ligaments, which are critical for sustaining long periods of running without injury.

You can include two days of strength training per week, focusing on bodyweight exercises such as squats, lunges, and planks, or weightlifting focusing on compound movements like deadlifts or bench press. Strengthening your core muscles is also vital as it contributes to better running form and endurance.

5.6. Don't Neglect Your Flexibility

Runners need a specific level of flexibility to maintain smooth and efficient running movements. Incorporating flexibility training in your weekly plan can help increase your range of motion, correct muscle imbalances, and reduce the risk of injury.

You could benefit from static stretches after your runs, dynamic stretches before your runs, and regular sessions of yoga or Pilates. This will help keep you supple and agile — critical attributes of any accomplished runner!

Train like a pro by adopting these practical workout plans into your routine. From race-specific training to strength exercises, maintaining a balance is crucial. Embrace the principles of consistency, intensity, and specificity in your training regime and don't forget the crucial role that flexibility and recovery play. Your finish line is just around the corner — faster and stronger than ever before!

Chapter 6. Interval Training: Speed Drills from the Fastest

Interval training has been a cornerstone in athletic training for over a century, and it's no less critical for today's elite runners. Its focus on achieving speed through structured, high-intensity workouts is essential for runners aiming to increase their pace and improve overall athletic performance.

The rationale behind interval training is compelling; it revolves around the concept of training physiological systems by periodically pushing them to their limits. Once these limits are identified and carefully stretched, the body adapts and makes necessary improvements, leading to enhanced speed and overall performance.

6.1. Understanding Interval Training

As the name suggests, interval training is composed of intervals or specific time periods in which you alternate high-intensity exercises with low-intensity recovery periods. These workouts are usually personalized to the runner's current performance level, targeting various energy systems within the body. From aerobic to anaerobic systems, each interval pushes a specific energy system to its limit to evoke the desired physiological adaptations.

Most importantly, interval training goes a long way in improving your VO2 max – which refers to the maximum amount of oxygen one can utilize during intense exercise. It's an indication of your endurance capacity and thus a useful measure for runners.

For example, a common interval training workout might comprise of running 400 meters at a high intensity, followed by a 200-meter jog or walk to recover - repeating this sequence several times.

6.2. Benefits of Interval Training

Interval training is far from a revolutionary concept. In fact, it constitutes the backbone of many training plans because it offers several benefits to athletes:

- Enhanced Aerobic Capacity: High-intensity interval training (HIIT) significantly elevates your maximal oxygen consumption (VO2 max), enhancing your aerobic capacity and subsequently, your running performance.

- Increased Lactate Threshold: Interval training can increase your body's ability to handle lactate accumulation during high-intensity efforts, allowing you to sustain these efforts for longer periods.

- Time-Efficiency: The high-intensity nature of interval training means that you'll receive significant results in shorter workout timeframes.

- Calorie Burn: Research indicates that interval training can result in higher post-exercise oxygen consumption, rendering it effective in calorie burning and weight management.

6.3. Designing an Interval Training Plan

Before delving into specific drills, it's worth noting that building an efficient interval training plan requires a thoughtful process. Just as essential as the workouts themselves is the approach that prioritizes gradual progression, individuality, and recovery.

To effectively design an interval training plan, the following steps should be kept in mind:

1. Establish your goals: Are you looking to improve race time, increase stamina, or build speed? The goals you set will consequently determine the type of intervals, their intensity and rest periods.

2. Assess current fitness level: Before designing a plan, have a realistic understanding of your current fitness level. This can be done using various metrics such as past race times or VO2 max.

3. Determine workout structure: The type of intervals (based on duration or intensity), rest or recovery between intervals, and the number of repetitions are pivotal components that form the workout structure.

4. Include Variety: Diversifying your interval training by encompassing a variety of exercises is beneficial in developing a more rounded athletic competence.

5. Track Your Progress: Reliable tracking can provide insightful feedback for recognizing improvement areas. Now, with numerous digital tools and wearables available, tracking, analyzing, and making adjustments couldn't be easier.

6.4. Speed Drills for Runners

Now, let's delve into some specific speed drills that are frequently incorporated in the training regimes of the fastest athletes in the world:

- **400-Meter Repeats**: This drill consists of running 400 meters at a high-intensity pace, then recovering at a slow jog or walk for the same distance. Repeat this sequence 8-10 times.

- **Hill Sprints**: Sprinting uphill recruits the large muscle groups in your legs, increasing their power and explosive speed while also improving your running stride. Sprint for 30 seconds uphill, then jog back down to recover.

- **Fartlek Runs**: The famed Swedish workout 'Fartlek' meaning 'speed play' is a flexible, unstructured form of interval training. It integrates varied paces throughout a normal run, and can consist of sprinting to the next mailbox, sprinting for a minute, or any other convenient measure.

- **Ladder Workouts**: These workouts involve running intervals of increasing or decreasing durations, with recovery in-between. The variety can engage multiple energy systems, offering comprehensive fitness improvements.

- **Tabata Training**: The Tabata protocol – composed of 20 seconds of all-out effort followed by 10 seconds of rest for a total of 4 minutes – can improve both your aerobic and anaerobic systems.

In conclusion, interval training is a potent tool to boost your speed, enhance overall race performance, and infuse some much-needed variety into your routine. However, remember to respect your body's need for recovery, to listen to its signals, and to gradually increase intensity. Always remember, increased performance results from a healthy balance between training stress and recovery. Happy running!

Chapter 7. Mastering the Art of Running Form and Technique

Before we delve into the precise biomechanics of running, it's important to underline that every runner has a unique style. A host of individual factors, such as body composition, flexibility, strength, natural rhythm, and even previous injury history, can influence your running style. That being said, understanding the fundamentals of efficient running form can provide standards against which you can assess your own technique and identify areas for improvement.

7.1. Principles of Efficient Running Form

When discussing running form, we must first understand the principles that underpin an efficient gait. The goal is not to mimic a certain style but to understand how movements and adjustments can conserve energy and minimize the risk of common running injuries.

- Forward lean: Efficient runners typically have a slight forward lean, originating from the ankles, not the hips. This forward lean uses gravity for propulsion, helping take some of the workload from the muscles.

- Arm swing: The arms should swing in a relaxed manner, with elbows bent at approximately 90 degrees. Arms should move front to back in a straight line, not across your body, and your hands should not cross the midline of your body.

- Footstrike: For most recreational runners, a midfoot strike (landing with the foot level to the ground) is recommended, as this reduces the forces sent back up into the body, which can reduce the risk of injuries.

<table>
<tr><td>NOTE</td><td>These principles are applicable for the majority of people, but always listen to your body. If a certain movement or adjustment feels uncomfortable or unnatural, it might not be suitable for you.</td></tr>
</table>

7.2. Running Cadence: The Metronome of Movement

Running cadence, the number of steps you take per minute, is another crucial facet of running form. An optimal cadence can help reduce the risk of injury and improve efficiency. The most commonly recommended cadence is roughly 180 steps per minute. To identify your running cadence, count the number of times your right foot hits the ground during a one-minute period, then double it. If you find your cadence is significantly lower than the suggested rate, look to gradually increase it over time.

7.3. Strength Training to Improve Form

Incorporating strength training into your routine can be an effective strategy to enhance running form. By focusing on exercises that extend your endurance and power, such as lunges, squats, or deadlifts, you can improve your hip, knee, and ankle flexibility and stability. Additionally, developing a strong core—encompassing your abs, lower back, and pelvic muscles—will support your overall running posture and stability.

7.4. Long Runs and Form Maintenance

Long runs are an integral part of any runner's training regimen. However, it's common to see technique falter as fatigue sets in. By focusing on your form throughout your long runs, you can improve your overall running technique.

7.5. Key Drills to Enhance Running Technique

By incorporating specific drills into your training, you can improve aspects of your running form. These exercises include high knee drives, butt kicks, and A-skips.

- High knee drives: These help to improve hip strength and flexibility, essential for powerful and efficient running.

- Butt kicks: These exercises focus on hamstring flexibility and speed.

- A-skips: These drills can help improve posture, rhythm, and footstrike.

7.6. Mental Role in Maintaining Running Form

Increasing your awareness of your running form and intentionally adjusting your movements to align with efficient running patterns can lead to noticeable improvements. It requires a measure of mindfulness and proactive engagement, as you must maintain focus on your body throughout your runs.

Running's repetitive nature can make it a meditative experience. By channeling your attention to your running form, this running "meditation" can be a powerful tool for improving your running economy.

7.7. Recovery and Form

Post-training recovery is just as important as the exercise itself when it comes to maintaining an efficient running form. This includes stretching, foam rolling, and taking rest days when they are needed.

By optimizing your running form and technique, you can not only boost your performance but also vastly reduce your risk of injuries. The compendium of insights shared in this chapter heralds the experience and wisdom of leading athletes, synthesized to give your running journey a substantial leap. Embrace these tips with open arms and conquer previously untouched frontiers of stamina, speed, and agility in your life as a runner.

Chapter 8. Cross-Training: Balancing Endurance and Strength

Strength and endurance form the two pillars of a successful runner's fitness regimen. On one hand, runners must perpetually boost their stamina to facilitate long-distance running, intervals, or sprints. On the contrary, it's equally crucial to build muscular strength for stability and speed. Therefore, cross-training—a training routine that blends various forms of exercise to ensure all-around athletic improvement—plays a cardinal role in ensuring a comprehensive approach, fostering a fine balance between endurance and strength.

8.1. Understanding Cross-Training

Cross-training acts as a buffer against monotony, injuries, and physical plateauing that might hinder your performance. Incorporating different types of exercises not only breaks the repetition of running but also aids in engaging various muscle groups, thus providing a well-rounded fitness routine. These alternate activities could range from weight lifting for strength, yoga for flexibility, to swimming or cycling for endurance enhancement.

8.2. The Role of Strength Training

Focusing on strength training is as crucial for runners as building endurance. These exercises help enhance muscle power, making it easier to propel oneself faster and with less effort.

Weight training and resistance exercises boost muscle strength and bone density, thereby augmenting a runner's speed and power. Additionally, strength training aids in maintaining a proper running form, even during bouts of exhaustion, thus diminishing the risks of sustaining injuries.

Begin with workouts targeting the major muscle groups such as the quadriceps, hamstrings, calf muscles, glutes, abdomen, and lower back. Squats, lunges, deadlifts, and calf raises are a few examples. You can progress towards more advanced workouts over time. It's essential to remember that resistance, rather than the number of repetitions, stimulates muscle growth and strength.

8.3. Incorporating Endurance Training

Endurance training is the fountainhead of a runner's fitness. It focuses on enhancing the body's ability to sustain prolonged periods of running without succumbing to fatigue. Two common forms of endurance training beneficial for runners are steady-state cardio and high-intensity interval training (HIIT).

1. **Steady-State Cardio:** This form of endurance training involves performing a low to moderate intensity exercise such as jogging or cycling for an extended period of time. These are great for active recovery days when you wish for a departure from robust running routines, yet aspire to work on your endurance.

2. **High-Intensity Interval Training (HIIT):** HIIT involves quick, intense bursts of exercise followed by short recovery periods. These intense workouts increase both your aerobic and anaerobic endurance, improving your ability to change pace rapidly during running. Exercises that can be part of your HIIT routine include bodyweight exercises such as burpees, mountain climbers, jumping jacks, or biking/sprinting at full throttle for brief periods.

8.4. The Advantages of Swimming and Cycling

Swimming and cycling emerge as beneficial cross-training exercises, offering a blend of strength and endurance workouts without adding stress to your joints, unlike running. Both these activities engage the cardiovascular system and strengthen the musculature simultaneously.

Swimming ensures a total body workout, engaging every major muscle group. It's particularly beneficial for strengthening the upper body, which is often less prioritized in a running regimen.

Cycling, on the other hand, helps runners build strong quads, glutes, and calves. Adopting a brisk cycling routine can boost your running pace and power.

8.5. Importance of Flexibility and Balance

In the quest for strength and endurance, it's easy to overlook flexibility and balance. However, these are components that ensure longevity in running. Yoga and Pilates can help improve body flexibility and balance. These create long, lean muscles that aid runners in maintaining form, enhancing speed, and preventing injuries.

Yoga also promotes mindfulness, an understated tool that helps you connect with your body better. With regular practice, runners may discern their body's signals better, which can be crucial during those rigorous marathon stretch-outs.

8.6. Conclusion

Cross-training implants diversity into your fitness regimen, endorsing a balanced workout routine that factors in not just your running prowess but overall athletic performance. By weaving workouts for strength and endurance with exercises to boost flexibility and balance, cross-training ensures a cohesive workout routine, keeping your body challenged and your spirits high. It's indeed a road less trod but one that undeniably leads to those coveted running milestones.

Chapter 9. Injury Prevention: Best Practices and Top Tips

Injury prevention is an indispensable part of any runner's training plan. It goes way beyond just "warming up" or "cooling down" – extending to comprehensive programs that cover strengthening activities, stretching exercises, diet plans, hydration, rest, and recovery. Understanding these aspects and incorporating them into your routine can dramatically reduce the risk of common running injuries. This chapter draws insights from top athletes and wellness experts to provide you with high-impact advice and best practices for injury prevention.

9.1. Understanding the Risk

Every runner, no matter how experienced, is at risk for certain injuries. These are usually due to overuse, incorrect form, inadequate nutrition, and insufficient recovery time. Overuse injuries, such as stress fractures and tendinitis, occur when runners push their bodies beyond their physical limits. They're often a result of escalating intensity, duration, or frequency of training too quickly. Understanding these risks is the first step to effective injury prevention.

1. Runners Knee, medically known as Patellofemoral Pain Syndrome, is the irritation of the cartilage on the underside of the kneecap. It may be caused by a poorly aligned kneecap, weak or imbalanced thigh muscles, or inadequate stretching.

2. Achilles Tendinitis is inflammation of the Achilles tendon, which connects the two major calf muscles to the back of the heel bone. It's mostly caused by rapid uphill or speed training.

3. Plantar Fasciitis is an inflammation of the band of tissue (the fascia) at the bottom of your foot that runs from your heel to your

toes. It's common in runners who have tight calf muscles, overpronate, or run excessive miles.

9.2. Strengthening Activities

Building strength, particularly in your leg and core muscles, is one of the best ways to reduce risk for running-related injuries. Strong muscles absorb impact forces better, thus helping to protect vulnerable tissues and joints.

Let's see three strengthening exercises recommended by top runners:

1. Squats: Squats target your quadriceps, hamstrings, and gluteal muscles, all of which are critical for running. They also engage your core, making them an excellent full-body exercise for runners.

2. Planks: Holding a plank position for an extended period strengthens your core muscles, which are crucial for maintaining good running form.

3. Calf raises: This move targets the often-overlooked calf muscles, which absorb a lot of impact during a run. Strong calves can help prevent a range of injuries, from shin splints to Achilles tendinitis.

9.3. Stretching Exercises

Stretching exercises increase flexibility and improve range of motion, reducing the risk of injuries. Keep in mind, stretching should never be painful. If you feel pain, you've gone too far.

1. Hamstring stretch: Lie on your back, keeping one knee bent. Take a strap or towel and loop it around the ball of your other foot. Slowly straighten your knee, feeling the stretch down the back of your leg.

2. Calf stretch: Stand in a lunge position with one leg forward and the other extended backward. Press your back heel into the ground until you feel a stretch in your calf muscle.

3. Quadriceps stretch: Stand on one leg. Grasp your ankle of the other leg and pull it up towards your rear. Keep your torso upright and feel the stretch in the front of your thigh.

9.4. Diet and Hydration

Your diet plays a significant role in preventing injuries. Following a diet high in antioxidants, and including ample amounts of protein, can help manage inflammation and promote recovery. Dehydration can also lead to muscle fatigue and cramps, increasing the risk of injuries. Therefore, ensure to drink plenty of water before, during, and after runs to stay adequately hydrated.

9.5. Rest and Recovery

Rest is equally crucial as training for preventing injuries. Overtraining without sufficient recovery time can lead to stress fractures, tendinitis, and other chronic ailments. Top athletes always ensure that their training plans include designated rest days. This allows their bodies to heal, reduce inflammation, and restore energy for the next session.

9.6. Listening to Your Body

Often, runners overlook early warning signs of injuries. A persistent discomfort or slight pain that doesn't resolve after a day or two could be a sign of an emerging problem. Listening to your body and backing off, or seeking medical advice when in doubt, is crucial in ensuring sustainable running.

Combining all these best practices — understanding risks,

strengthening and stretching exercises, proper diet, hydration, rest and recovery, and listening to your body — will give you a comprehensive injury prevention strategy. Remember, the best runners in the world didn't achieve their prowess overnight. They put in consistent, mindful effort, patiently building their endurance, speed, and resilience while taking steps to prevent injuries. With this in-depth insight into injury prevention, you're now equipped to carry forward your running passion in a sustainable and healthier manner!

Chapter 10. Mindset and Motivation: Harnessing Mental Stamina

Mindset and motivation have paramount importance in sport, especially in running, where individuals often have to feud against their own limitations rather than an external adversary. Harnessing mental stamina is a skill; the good news is, like any other skill, it can be honed and refined over time.

10.1. The Power of Mindset

Your mindset is the lens through which you perceive the world around you. It is a subtle, often overlooked aspect, but it can have a profound impact on your running performance. There are two types of mindsets: fixed and growth. People with a fixed mindset believe that their abilities are set in stone and cannot change, which results in avoiding challenges and giving up easily. In contrast, those with a growth mindset regard challenges as opportunities to learn and improve. They believe they can get better with effort and persistence over time.

It is crucial for runners to possess a growth mindset. If you believe you can improve and you're willing to put work into it, you're in a much better position to surpass your limitations.

10.2. Developing a Growth Mindset

Switching from a fixed to a growth mindset won't happen overnight. It takes time, dedication, and conscious effort. Here are a few strategies to help you develop a growth mindset.

1. Identify your fixed mindset traps: Being self-aware can help you realize when you're falling into a fixed mindset. You can then consciously decide to switch your thinking.

2. Embrace failure and learning: Failures are stepping stones on the path to success. Look at every shortcoming as a learning opportunity.

3. Keep the mantra of "Efforts over Outcomes": Focus on the effort you're putting into your training and improvement, rather than just the outcome of races or time trials.

10.3. Building Mental Stamina

Mental stamina entails your capacity for sustained attention, cognitive effort, and enduring emotional resilience. Enhanced mental stamina doesn't just lead to better performance; it also promotes faster recovery and improved overall well-being.

Here are some strategies to build mental stamina:

1. Emotional Regulation: Practice managing your emotions when the going gets tough. Meditation, mindfulness, or Cognitive Behavioural Therapy (CBT) techniques can be beneficial.

2. Mental Imagery: Use your imagination to create scenarios in your mind that help you tackle challenging situations. Practice positive visualization techniques regularly.

3. Goal Setting: Having clear, attainable goals gives you a sense of purpose and a clear direction. Set SMART (Specific, Measurable, Achievable, Relevant, Time-bound) goals.

4. Self-Talk: The language you use for yourself matters. Make sure it's positive, encouraging, and motivating.

10.4. Tapping into Intrinsic Motivation

Intrinsic motivation comes from within you. It's about engaging in behavior because you enjoy it and find it inherently satisfying. This is remarkably significant for runners, as a love for running can keep you moving when the going gets tough.

A few ways to tap into your intrinsic motivation include:

1. Stay Curious: Always be open to learning. Appreciate the process and every stride you take towards improvement.

2. Play: Make running fun. Join running groups, participate in different races, or explore new routes.

3. Autonomy: Take ownership of your running journey. You're the boss of your progress and your choices.

4. Competence: Feel competent about what you do. Celebrate your small victories.

Running is an exceptional journey, one which can teach a soul more about themselves and the world than they ever imagined. The lessons of discipline, resilience, and perseverance often bleed into other areas of life, making runners stronger, not just physically, but also mentally. So harness your mental stamina, wear your running shoes, and let the journey start!

In the next chapter, we will delve deeper into the nuts and bolts of a runner's nutrition and its impact on performance. We hope this stamina steeled exploration has strengthened your resolve to improve your running journey. Enjoy the run!

Chapter 11. Recovery Secrets: Understanding the Role of Rest and Sleep

Running is not just about the distance covered or the time clocked; it's equally about the time spent recovering and rejuvenating. A finely tuned recovery regimen can make the difference between a runner who consistently improves and one who gets stuck in an endless cycle of injuries or performance plateaus.

11.1. The Importance of Rest and Recovery

Every stride you take on a run leads to some degree of muscle damage, cellular breakdown, and glycogen depletion. Rest periods allow the body to self-repair this harm and improvise on these physiological abilities, thereby enhancing endurance, speed, and strength incrementally. This down-time is when actual growth happens, when muscles heal and get stronger.

Typically, there are two key recovery components: Rest, which simply implies giving oneself a break from running, and sleep, an often-underestimated yet vital part of the process. Both encompass a wider set of practices, including nutrition and mental relaxation.

Running concurrently with inadequate rest can lead to overuse injuries like shin splints, tendonitis, and stress fractures. It may also result in overtraining syndrome accompanied by signs like increased fatigue, decreased performance, or aggravated mood swings. The need for adequate rest cannot be stressed enough, making it an indispensable part of your training regimen.

Rest is the body's chance to adapt to training stresses, repair tissues, and replenish glycogen stores. These adaptive processes are driven by an array of hormones and metabolic functions, which reach their peak during periods of adequate rest.

The hormone responsible for the majority of adaptive responses, particularly muscle repair and development, is human growth hormone (HGH). This is released in abundance during deep, restful periods and is key to muscle recovery and strength increases.

Another hormone crucial for rest and recovery is cortisol. This hormone aids in the regulation and mobilisation of energy during intense exercise. During periods of rest, cortisol levels decrease, allowing the body to replenish energy stores and mend any damaged tissues.

11.2. Rest Day: Passive versus Active

There are two primary categories of rest: passive and active. Passive rest symbolizes complete cessation from running and any strenuous physical activity. This type of rest is significant intermittently during training cycles or after a major race.

Active rest, on the other hand, refers to light cross-training exercises that keep the blood flowing but don't chalk up to additional stress on the body. Swimming, cycling, and yoga are superb examples of active rest activities that grant immense physiological and psychological benefits without derailing the recovery process.

11.3. Sleep: The Elixir of Recovery

While periods of conscious rest are critical, nothing quite compares to the impact of nocturnal slumber on recovery. Sleep is the body's primary recovery tool, providing physiological and psychological healing like none other.

==| The Science of Sleep

During sleep, several vital processes come into play. The pineal gland releases melatonin, a hormone that regulates sleep-wake cycles. This release contributes to the reparative work carried out during sleep, including the healing and growth of cells and the consolidation of memories and learning.

Rapid Eye Movement (REM) sleep, which accounts for about 20-25% of the total sleep in adults, is considered crucial for learning and memory. Slow Wave Sleep (SWS), the deep sleep stage, initiates increased release of growth hormone, further promoting repair and growth processes.

An optimal balance between REM sleep and SWS is vital for runners. It allows for cognitive functions related to decision-making, reaction time, and emotional well-being while also promoting tissue repair and efficient energy metabolism.

11.4. Sleep Hygiene: Optimizing your Sleep

Sleep is indeed essential, but quality sleep is truly pivotal. With improving sleep getting mainstream attention, we have now coined the term 'sleep hygiene.' This term corresponds to practices that promote better, deeper, and more restful sleep.

Here are some strategies even top runners swear by:

1. Regularity: A consistent sleep schedule, even on off days, elevates your sleep quality.
2. Environment: Dark, cool, and silent environments are most

conducive to sound sleep.

3. Pre-sleep routine: A consistent pre-sleep routine signals your body about impending bedtime.

4. Nutrition: Avoiding large meals, caffeine, alcohol, and nicotine close to bedtimes can significantly improve sleep quality.

It's essential to continuously assess and modify your rest and sleep routines to benefit maximally. This is because your body's recovery capability changes with increased training load, age, and life stressors. Understanding your body and adjusting your rest and recovery strategies is the best approach to sustain long-term running health.

As we weave through the myriad of strategies available, remember, everyone is unique. It's crucial for you to listen to your body and determine what blend of rest and sleep works best for your regime. After all, the path to performance improvement isn't about punishing your body, but about training smarter. Rest easy, knowing that by setting aside time for recovery, you're truly investing in your running progression.

Remember to mix in elements of both active and passive rests as per your body's need and never compromise on the quality of your sleep. In addition to these, a balanced diet and controlled mental stress play an equal role in enabling effective recovery. After all, running isn't just about the miles or the effort — it's about the journey, and learning to pace ourselves for the long run is what makes us better athletes.

www.ingramcontent.com/pod-product-compliance
Lightning Source LLC
Chambersburg PA
CBHW070743260726

48660CB00007B/2956